"Unveiling Nourish: A Deep Dive into the Gavelston Diet Revolution"

Copyright

Table Of Contents

Introduction

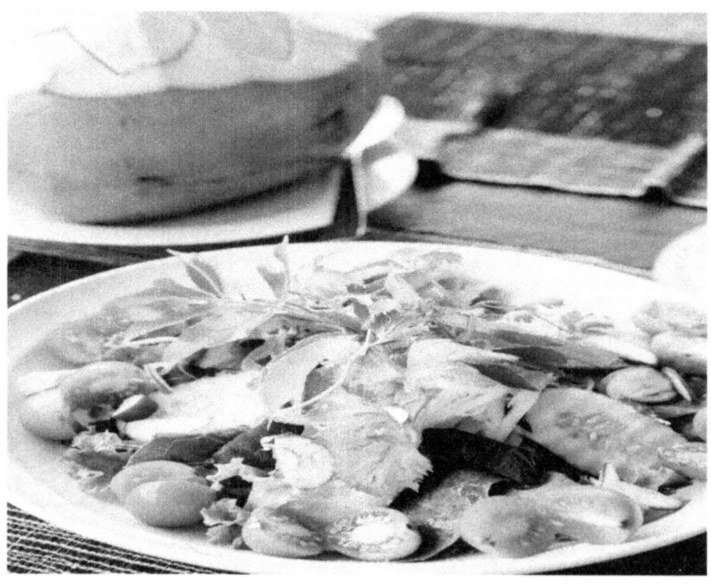

The Gavelston diet, which takes its name from the picturesque seaside village of Gavelston, has become well-known for its all-encompassing approach to health and nutrition. This diet plan, which is based on the idea of balance, places an emphasis on the harmonious blending of whole foods that are produced locally and attentive eating habits.

Fundamentally, the Gavelston diet avoids processed foods, high sugar content, and chemical additives and places an emphasis on lean meats, fresh, organic veggies, and healthy fats. Its emphasis on individualized meal plans that take into account lifestyle, health objectives, and dietary preferences sets it apart from other diets.

The Gavelston diet celebrates a wide variety of nutrient-dense foods by incorporating a vivid array of flavors and textures that are inspired by Mediterranean and Asian culinary traditions.

In addition to its nutritional components, the Gavelston diet encourages a balanced lifestyle that includes frequent exercise, plenty of fluids, and enough sleep.

The Gavelston diet seeks to improve overall well-being by encouraging good, sustainable eating practices. It assists people in reaching their health goals and builds a long-lasting relationship with nourishing, delectable food options.

Chapter 1 . The Issue

What's glucose once more

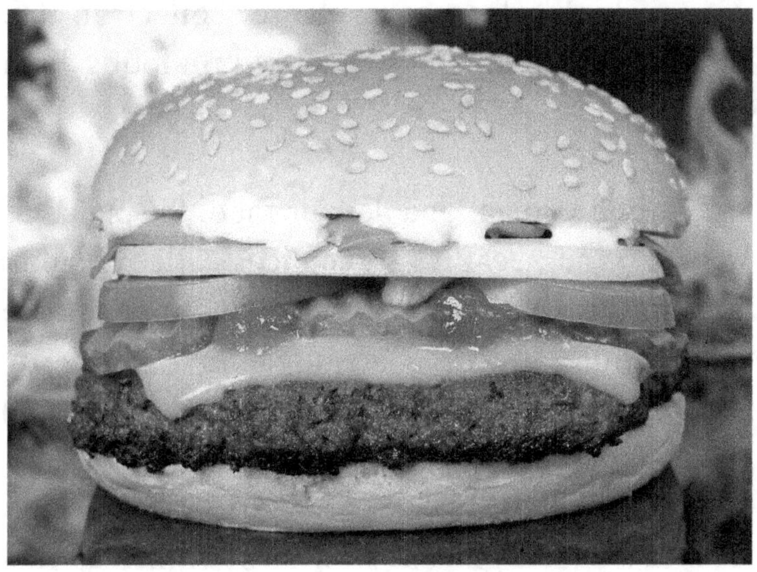

The human body is a mind boggling machine that is defenseless to numerous infections and conditions that can hamper it.

High glucose and weight gain or misfortune are by a wide margin two of the most notable and most normal circumstances that have been ailing the human species however long we know.

Glucose, a sort of sugar, is the primary wellspring of energy in the body. At the point when an individual has diabetes, his/her body can't deal with glucose appropriately. This causes high glucose levels to collect in the circulation system subsequently prompting high glucose.

Each time you eat and devour food, the pancreas delivers and secretes a chemical called insulin. Insulin assists the body with handling glucose and bridle energy acquired by food by essentially helping to move the glucose (sugar) inside every cell for the creation of energy.

The embedded glucose is what's utilized as fuel to make energy for your body. In diabetes, there is either less creation or insulin of an obstruction made towards insulin relying upon the sort of diabetes you have.

Because of the infectivity of insulin, the glucose got from the utilization of food in the event that it was not sent into the cells. This makes the sugar stay in the blood accordingly bringing about high glucose levels in the circulatory system. This state of having overabundance sugar in the blood is high glucose.

Diabetes And Its Connection To Weight Gain
Diabetes is by a long shot quite possibly the most uncontrolled clinical infirmity that has spread across the globe.

Frequently, contingent upon the sort of diabetes, individuals find that they either gain or get more fit definitely while experiencing diabetes. Type-2 diabetes is the reason for weight gain in the stomach.

Numerous patients have had issues concerning weight gain even before the settlement of diabetes in them.

Individuals who are overweight and fat have a much higher gamble of creating diabetes in later phases of their life when contrasted with others. Likewise, the people who have diabetes and have left it undiscovered for a while can likewise find an expansion in their weight.Diabetes doesn't prompt the acquiring of weight and heftiness straightforwardly. However, patients who have been experiencing uncontrolled diabetes before would, truth be told, put on weight as the glucose level in the blood would standardize. This is ordinarily viewed as the recovering of recently shed pounds.

Extra people can foster heftiness and weight gain because of indulging. Indulging is viewed as an ordinary indication of patients with diabetes as they go into hypoglycemia because of ill-advised treatment.

The patient might show just long for low glucose (hypoglycemia) and no other such side effects. There are likewise a couple of hostile to diabetic medications that when recommended, may prompt weight gain.

side effects and conditions connected with glucose spike

At times, it is feasible to direct blood glucose levels through way of life changes. Notwithstanding, certain individuals might require prescriptions.

The pancreas secretes a chemical called insulin that makes cells more delicate to glucose. The cells then, at that point, draw glucose from the blood, lessening the impacts of glucose spikes.

In an individual with diabetes, either the pancreas doesn't deliver insulin or the cells foster a protection from this chemical. Subsequently, the glucose stays in the blood, keeping glucose levels reliably high. This is called hyperglycemia.

In individuals living with diabetes, glucose spikes frequently happen in the wake of eating. Overall, this happens 75 minutes after the beginning of dinner.

Notwithstanding, on the off chance that an individual can't deal with their condition, they might have constant high blood glucose levels. This can prompt entanglements of diabetes, including nerve harm, vision misfortune, kidney harm, kidney issues, and an expanded gamble of cardiovascular sickness.

High glucose (hyperglycemia) is normal in individuals with type 1 or type 2 diabetes however it can likewise happen in individuals without these illnesses. The reasons for glucose ascending in a nondiabetic incorporate a significant disease, a persistent ailment, a hormonal issue, or certain medications. Your family ancestry and hereditary qualities likewise may add to nondiabetic hyperglycemia. So can specific way of life factors, similar to eating less and your degree of exercise. The measure of glucose in the circulatory system is directed by insulin, a chemical delivered by the pancreas. After a dinner, insulin will close down the arrival of glucose from the liver to guarantee levels don't get excessively high.

At the point when any of these frameworks are weakened — including the various organs that direct the pancreas — glucose can be delivered improperly and cause high glucose. It can likewise happen in the event that liver cells become less receptive with the impacts of insulin, known as insulin opposition.

Nondiabetic hyperglycemia might happen as a preface to diabetes —, for example, with prediabetes (disabled glucose resistance) — or it might have no relationship to diabetes at all. Contingent upon the seriousness of the case, side effects of high glucose without diabetes include:

1. Cerebral pains
2. Expanded thirst or appetite
3. Incessant pee (peeing)
4. Extreme exhaustion
5. Obscured vision
6. Quick pulses
7. Shivering, consuming, or deadness in your grasp or feet

8. Incessant diseases or slow-mending wounds

Normal Reasons for Nondiabetic Hyperglycemia

There are five(5) normal reasons for nondiabetic hyperglycemia that straightforwardly or in a roundabout way disturb the connection between the pancreas (which produces insulin) and the liver (which produces glucose).

A. Cushing's Condition

Cushing's condition is a problem brought about by the overabundant discharge of adrenocorticotropic chemical (ACTH) delivered by the pituitary organ. This, thus, makes the adrenal organs produce extreme measures of cortisol, the body's fundamental pressure chemical.

When a lot of cortisol is delivered, it can balance the impacts of insulin and lead to insulin obstruction. It can likewise diminish how much insulin is delivered by the pancreas.

B. Injury

Actual pressure to the body, including injury, consumes, and different wounds, can cause high glucose by modifying how glucose is used. An investigation of in excess of 95,000 individuals observed that this condition was related with an expanded gamble of death following an injury occurrence.

C. Stress-instigated hyperglycemia

This happens when the body's instinctive reaction sets off the arrival of cortisol and one more pressure chemical known as epinephrine (adrenaline). Epinephrine expands the creation of glucose, while glucose obstructs the impacts of insulin.

Medical procedure and Stress

Modifications to glucose digestion that happen from actual pressure to the body likewise happen after a medical procedure. Medical procedure is a controlled type of pressure to the body that results in comparative expansions in cytokines and chemicals that drive the development of glucose in the liver and block the impacts of insulin from eliminating overabundance glucose from the blood.

Up to 30% of individuals can foster pressure instigated hyperglycemia after medical procedure, with blood glucose levels that stay raised long subsequent to getting back from the clinic. Raised glucose after medical procedure can altogether affect generally speaking wellbeing and expands the gamble of creating diabetes and other difficult circumstances.

D. Heftiness

High glucose is related with heftiness since abundance fat cells upset the equilibrium of glucose and insulin.9 Overabundance fat cells called adipocytes discharge provocative proteins, for example, interleukins and growth putrefaction factor, which increment the body's protection from insulin by enacting processes that disturb the body's capacity to deliver and deliver insulin when glucose is high.

Overabundance fat cells likewise decline the capacity to eliminate glucose from the blood to be utilized for energy or put away as glycogen inside skeletal muscles. With heftiness, expanded lipids, or unsaturated fat particles, actuate pathways that debilitate insulin motioning inside muscles.

E. Hereditary qualities

A family background of diabetes can build your gamble of creating hyperglycemia. While diabetes can be forestalled through diet and way of life factors, disabled insulin responsiveness can run in families and may make you more inclined to growing high glucose.

Pregnant individuals can likewise foster gestational diabetes, frequently somewhere in the range of 24 and 28 weeks of pregnancy, because of hormonal changes that influence how glucose is used in the body. The impact of pregnancy chemicals can impede the capacity of insulin to eliminate overabundance glucose from the blood, causing glucose to remain raised.

Menopause can cause a huge change in chemicals, weight, and body creation. The Galveston diet looks to reestablish this disturbed hormonal equilibrium while assisting you with keeping a steady weight. The accentuation on calming dinners, supplement rich cancer prevention agent stacked food varieties, and part control makes this diet stand apart from different methodologies. It centers around creating smart dieting propensities that are not difficult to support. This eating plan could simply be the ticket for the smooth wellness venture you were sitting tight for.

Chapter 2 .A way out

History of the gavelston diet

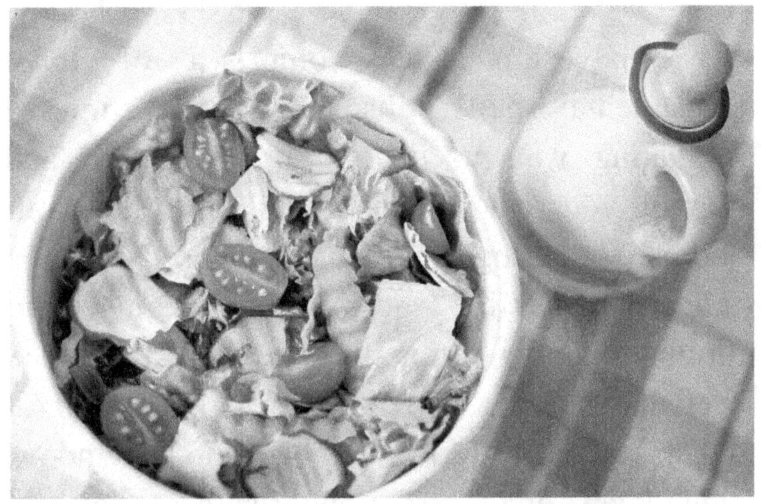

The Galveston Diet was intended for ladies in all periods of menopause, including perimenopause, who need to keep away from weight gain and might be attempting to shed pounds during these phases of life. It can likewise assist with normal hormonal side effects like hot blazes, night sweats, and mind haze. Dr. Mary Claire Haver, an OBGYN doctor, made the Galveston Diet to assist individuals with menopause get thinner. The premise of the Galveston Diet is a mitigating way to deal with nourishment and discontinuous fasting.

The Galveston Diet comprises of three fundamental parts: discontinuous fasting, a mitigating way to deal with sustenance, and moving your wholesome admission to fuel your body, The eating routine is supposed to be a calming diet like the Mediterranean eating routine yet additionally incorporates 16:8 irregular fasting," (FYI: That is the point at which you eat during an eight-hour window, then keep away from nourishment for the leftover 16 hours of the day.) "The eating routine cutoff points handled food varieties that contain added sugar, counterfeit fixings, varieties and flavorings, white flour, food sources with high-fructose corn syrup, liquor, seared food sources, and vegetable oils."

What are you permitted to eat on the Galveston Diet?

There are bunches of heavenly food varieties you can integrate into the Galveston Diet, including the following:

- Fruits (lower in sugar): Strawberries, blueberries and raspberries.
- Vegetables (low in starch): Greens, tomatoes, cucumbers, celery, zucchini, broccoli.
- Lean proteins: Chicken, salmon, fish, turkey, eggs.
- Vegetables: Beans (chickpeas, dark beans), lentils, nuts and seeds (pecans, almonds, chia seeds).
- Entire grains: Entire wheat bread, earthy colored rice, quinoa, grain, oats, buckwheat.
- Dairy: Milk, yogurt, cheddar.
- Sound fats: Olive oil, avocado oil.

What food sources are not permitted on the Galveston Diet?

The Galveston Diet urges you to avoid food varieties that are favorable to incendiary and need dietary benefit, which can cause weight gain and pose little advantage to your general wellbeing. You're most likely currently acquainted with in any event a portion of these.

What are the upsides and downsides of the Galveston Diet?

The Galveston Diet doesn't expect you to count calories, which might turn out better for certain individuals. Furthermore, the eating routine spotlights on assisting you with creating good dieting and exercise propensities that will put you in a good position over the long haul as opposed to confining and crash dieting.If you're new to the 16:8 eating regimen, it might forestall late-evening eating or nibbling. On the other side, it might make certain individuals indulge during the taking care of window to forestall sensations of appetite some other time when they shouldn't eat.Also, you can change the Galveston

Diet with the goal that it works for plant-based eaters. "It tends to be made veggie lover or vegetarian agreeable, yet the eating regimen itself doesn't kill creature based food sources,"
numerous ladies who attempted this diet accomplished their weight reduction objectives and felt better and more sure than previously.

Also, the eating routine is protected. Simply try to check in with your doctor prior to making a plunge, particularly in the event that you're immunosuppressed or have diabetes or a background marked by scattered eating on the grounds that discontinuous fasting isn't prescribed if any of these concerns you.

How gavelston diet works
The Galveston eating plan includes three significant activities:

1. Stay away from Provocative Food varieties
Food varieties said to add to irritation in the body are confined to this arrangement.

aggravation advancing toll incorporates sugars, handled grains, broiled food sources, handled lunch meats, immersed fats, and sodaInstead, the eating routine stresses entire food varieties with bunches of non starchy vegetables and natural products.

Food varieties explicitly accepted to decrease irritation are energized, like greasy fish, berries, garlic, nuts, tomatoes, and olive oil.

2. Practice Irregular Fasting

The thought is that an extended length of time between dinners makes your cells more versatile to stressors and furthermore starts significant cell fix.

The kind of irregular fasting (IF) suggested in the Galveston diet is known as 16/8, and that implies fasting for 16 hours and eating during a window of 8 hours consistently. That for the most part implies deferring the principal feast of the day until around early afternoon.

With regards to menopausal ladies, there has been some worry that discontinuous fasting could influence chemical levels, yet a review distributed in the diary Stoutness in October 2022 tried twelve postmenopausal ladies (as well as twelve premenopausal ladies) following two months of a considerably stricter eating windows of four to six hours. It tracked down no progressions in degrees of estrone, testosterone, and most other sex chemicals.

3. Up Your Fat Consumption

Contrasted and the commonplace American eating regimen, the Galveston diet slices carbs decisively. Here, the main part of calories — exactly 70% right away — come from solid fats. To support fat consumption, this change in energy obtained is designated "fuel pulling together."

"The point is to accomplish an ideal proportion of fat to protein to starch that advances fat misfortune in the fat-misfortune stage,"

Proteins make up the following biggest piece of the eating regimen, with supplement thick starches the littlest part.

After you've been on the eating regimen for some time and you become accustomed to eating less carbs and sugars, some extra complicated carbs are placed in.

The Galveston diet primarily works by advancing the utilization of good food sources like entire grains, verdant green vegetables and organic products, and sound fats. The eating routine additionally puts itself in a good position due to how maintainable it is over the long haul. The spotlight isn't such a great amount on eating less for all intents and purposes on eating a greater amount of the great stuff. Loads of handled meats like bacon and hotdogs, as well as sweet beverages, refined grains like white bread and pasta, and seared food varieties energize irritation in the body. Removing those can be incredibly helpful to general wellbeing.

Eating food varieties that further develop irritation markers in our bodies likewise influences our stomach, which thus influences our mind-set. As we progress in years, our bodies battle to process food appropriately in view of changes in insulin responsiveness and a more slow digestion. The solid eating routine supported by the Galveston program settles insulin levels as well.

Advantages of the Gavelston diet

1. May Assist with decreasing Weight
A few examinations have noticed the gainful impacts of irregular fasting on weight on the board. It can lessen 0.8% to 13% of body weight and abatement your weight index by a normal of 4.3%. No serious secondary effects, other than cravings for food, were accounted for

While water misfortune adds to the underlying weight reduction saw on a low-carb diet, genuine fat decrease happens when one sticks to this kind of diet in the long haul

2. May Diminish Ongoing Irritation

Aggravation is your invulnerable framework's normal reaction to injury or disease. Be that as it may, constant aggravation has been connected to a few medical issue like diabetes, coronary illness, and specific sorts of malignant growth

Irregular fasting brings down incendiary signals and forestalls the obstructing of veins. This brings down the gamble of a few cardiovascular problems. Moreover, studies propose that low-carb diets might assist with diminishing irritation and lighten conditions like Parkinson'si , various sclerosis , and greasy liver infection

3. May Assist with controlling Glucose.

A few investigations recommend that embracing an exceptionally low-starch ketogenic diet and transforming one's way of life can work on the strength of individuals who are overweight and have type 2 diabetes. Be that as it may, not all results were indisputable as certain subjects showed insulin resistance while others worked on their awareness towards the chemical through this eating routine. Consequently, further long haul studies are justified in such a manner.

4. Doesn't Count Calories

Counting calories can cause pressure when you are attempting to adhere to a severe calorie limit. However, staying away from it can lessen pressure and further develop your general prosperity. As opposed to zeroing in on the quantity of calories you eat, you can zero in on the healthy benefit of the food.

Inflexibly counting calories can prompt disordered eating designs like pigging out, limitation, and fixation. Zeroing in on food quality rather than amount can decrease the gamble of disarranged eating.

Not including calories doesn't mean you ought to overlook the energy equilibrium of what you are eating. All things considered, center around supplementing thick and fulfilling food sources and permit yourself a periodic treat. Continue to peruse to more deeply study the food sources you can have on this eating routine.

Other advantages

Alongside decreasing body weight, the Galveston Diet might have other medical advantages, because of its mitigating approach and irregular fasting strategies.

May lessen irritation

As per a 2020 reviewTrusted Source, discontinuous fasting lessens irritation in the body that emerges from fat tissue (fat stores).

A similar report likewise demonstrates that irregular fasting might attempt to forestall insulin opposition and diabetes.

May decrease chance of specific illnesses

A 2021 reviewTrusted Source proposes the useful mitigating impacts of discontinuous fasting may likewise assist with forestalling constant circumstances like metabolic disorder and cardiovascular illness.

Discontinuous fasting may likewise check the harming impacts of oxidative pressure, which produces free revolutionaries that cause illness and maturing.

A 2019 survey reasoned that irregular fasting could assist with forestalling hypertension and conditions, for example, malignant growth as well as draw out life expectancy.

May further develop inspiration
The additional help and action components of some Galveston Diet program memberships might imply that individuals attempting the eating regimen feel more roused to stay with it. Additionally, they might lead people to participate in more active work than they typically do. Both of these things might help weight reduction and general wellbeing.

Is the Gavelston diet for you

The eating regimen is explicitly intended for individuals in the perimenopausal and menopausal periods, although it could be useful for ladies as youthful as 35.

To make it work for you, it is prescribed to take on the progressions suggested by the eating regimen gradually "with an end goal to assemble new propensities that will endure and to stay away from overpower."

It Proposes that ladies keep a receptive outlook about the Galveston diet. "At the point when you hit midlife, your requirements are explicit, "Your body is changing and it's not difficult to get anxious with yourself. You may not move results immediately, however that is important for the regular course of maturing."

Chapter 3. Getting everything rolling

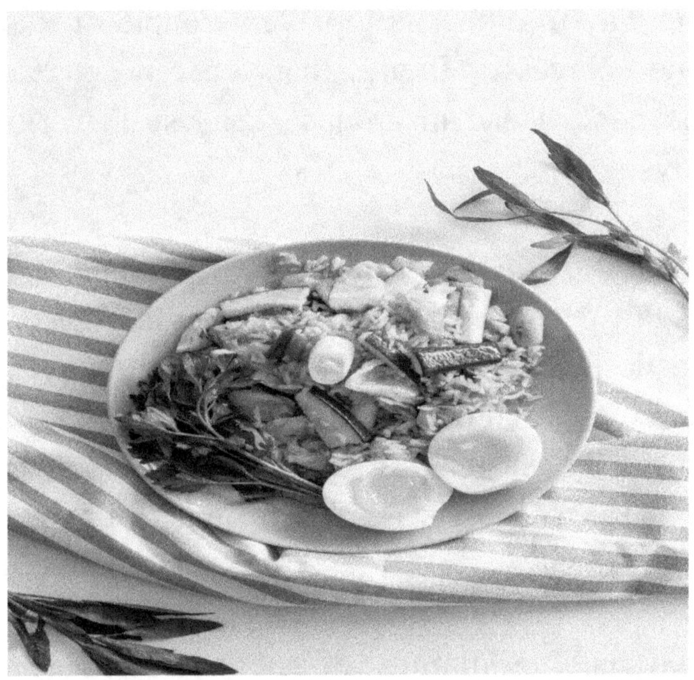

Knowing what to eat, the amount to eat, when to eat, and afterward setting up your feasts is one of the main parts of accomplishing a sound, adjusted diet. The Galveston Diet centers around calming sustenance: restricting openness to additives and synthetic substances and handling sugars and stacking up on natural products, veggies, lean protein, and fiber.

The way to dinner is to have a couple of staple food sources or fixings that you can get ready and cook ahead in groups, then use in various ways.

My 6 Top Dinner Prep Tips:
A. Put resources into a lot of reusable glass or plastic holders and zip-top packs - they're your new closest companion and are critical to your prosperity. Search for partitioned compartments - these will assist with keeping your feasts coordinated.

B. Intend to diminish waste and keep feasts fascinating. Put your family down and make an arrangement together - so everybody is locked in and amped up for the weeks' feasts. Begin little when you initially start dinner preparing. Find a central arrangement of recipes your family loves - in a matter of moments, you will have them remembered, making this try so natural!

C. Make a shopping list - and stick to it.

Cook in enormous clusters and freeze or refrigerate for feasts during the week. Have no-cook, in and out things close by - organic products, slashed veggies, and nuts to toss into holders.

Put away a couple of hours every week to slash and cook - it will save you hours over the long haul. In our family, Sunday is feast prep day!

D. Place berries and slashed veggies in an enormous partitioned compartment, making in and out for your family simple for eating or tossing into holders!

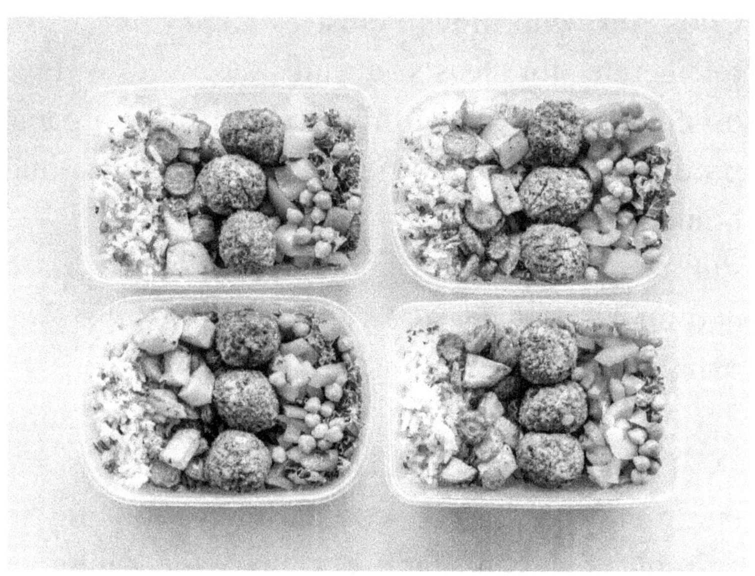

1. Spinach and goat cheddar omelet
Ingredients

- 3 eggs
- 2 haze ladles(30 mL) of weighty cream
- 1 mug(30 grams) of spinach
- 1 ounce(28 grams) of goat cheddar
- 1 tablespoon(14 grams) of spread tar and pepper to taste

Procedures

Whisk the eggs, weighty cream, tar, and pepper in a bowl, also put the combination down. run the margarine in a skillet over medium intensity and sauté the spinach. Mix infrequently until the spinach is dim green and withered. barred from the vessel and put down. Empty the egg combination into the dish and cook it over medium intensity. When the eggs begin to set, flip them over exercising a spatula. Add spinach and goat cheddar to half of the omelet. When the omelet has set, crinkle it down the middle and serve.

2. Veggie frittata

Ingredients

- 6 eggs mug(80 mL) of milk tar and pepper to taste
- 4 cloves of garlic, minced
- mugs(60 grams) of kale,
- slashed mugs(300 grams) of chime peppers,
- slashed ounce(28 grams) of disintegrated feta

- 1 tablespoon(15 mL) of olive oil

Procedures

Preheat the range to 400 °F(205 °C). Whisk the eggs, milk, minced garlic, tar, and pepper, also put the combination down. Add the olive oil painting oil to a 10- inch(25- cm), range safe skillet over medium intensity. Sauté the addressed kale and ringer peppers, mixing apropos until mellowed, or around 5- 7 beats. Pour in the egg blend and slant the skillet to equitably convey it. Sprinkle the feta over the top. Prepare 15- 20 beats in the skillet until the eggs are set, also season, cut, and serve.

3. toast avocado eggs

Ingredients

- 1 avocado
- 2 eggs
- salt and pepper to taste
- voluntary beautifiers, like bacon bits, cheddar, chives, cilantro, or tomatoes

Procedures

Preheat the toaster oven to 400 °F(205 °C). Cut the avocado fifty, including the hole, and use a spoon to lade out a portion from the center and make the opening lower. Break one egg into each opening. Season with tar, pepper, and add your selection of beautifiers. Heat for 10- 15 beats and serve.

4. Shakshuka

Ingredients

- 6 eggs
- 1 onion
- Diced red ringer pepper,
- Diced cloves of garlic, minced
- a 28- ounce(794- gram) jar of squashed tomatoes
- Salt and pepper to taste
- 1 tablespoon(7 grams) of paprika
- teaspoon(1 gram) of red bean stew cream
- 1 teaspoon(2 grams) of cumin
- 2 ounces(57 grams) of feta
- 1 pack of cilantro

Procedures

Add oil to a vessel over medium intensity. Sauté diced onions and ringer peppers for 3- 5 beats, or until the onions turn clear. Empty the canned tomatoes into the vessel with juice. Mix in the minced garlic, tar, pepper, and flavors and carry the combination to a stew. exercising a spoon, make 6 little openings in the blend and break 1 egg into each. Cover the vessel and cook for 5-10 beats, or until the eggs have arrived at your ideal degree of doneness. Top with feta and cilantro and serve.

5. Broccoli and bacon crustless quiche
Ingredients
- 6 eggs
- 1 mug(240 mL) of milk
- 1 mug(90 grams) of broccoli
- slashed cuts of bacon
- 4 mug(85 grams) of cheddar
- 2 haze ladles(30 mL) of olive oil
- Salt and pepper to taste

Procedures

Preheat the range to 350 °F(180 °C). Cook the bacon in a vessel over medium intensity for 5- 10 beats, or until establishment. Put it to the side on a kerchief- lined plate. Add the olive oil to the dish and sauté the stuck broccoli for 3- 4 beats. Circulate the broccoli and bacon slightly at the lower part of a lubed 9- inch(23- cm) pie dish. In a little bowl, whisk the eggs, milk, tar, and pepper. Pour the egg combination over the pie dish and outdo it with cheddar. Heat for 30- 35 beats until the eggs have set. Cool and serve.

6. Zoodle egg holmes

Ingredients

- 2 zucchinis
- spiralized eggs
- 1 tablespoon(30 mL) of olive oil
- Salt and pepper to taste
- voluntary seasoning

Procedures

Cut avocado, or red pepper pieces captions Preheat the oven to 350 °F(180 °C). Add the olive oil to a skillet and sauté the zucchini over medium intensity for 2- 3 beats, or until delicate. Arrange each spiralized zucchini in a skillet to make a holme. Break an egg in the middle, sprinkle with swab and pepper, and heat for 5 beats. Add wanted beautifiers and serve.

7. Veggie egg mugs

Ingredients

- 12 eggs
- mug(80 mL) of milk
- mug(29 grams) of red onion, diced
- mug(70 grams) of mushrooms, diced
- mug(150 grams) of ringer peppers, diced
- 1/ 2 mug(90 grams) of tomatoes
- mug(110 grams) of cheddar
- 2 haze ladles(30 mL) of olive oil
- Salt and pepper to taste

Procedures

Preheat the toaster oven to 350 °F(180 °C). Add the olive oil to a skillet and sauté the vegetables over medium intensity for 5 beats, or until mellowed. lade the vegetables and cheddar equitably into a lubed, 12- mug biscuit barrel. In a little bowl, blend the eggs, milk, tar, and pepper. Circulate the blend also into each mug of the biscuit barrel. Prepare for 20- 25 beats, or until set, and cool former to serving.

8. Fried eggs with wiener
Ingredients
- 2 eggs
- 2 haze ladles(30 mL) of weighty cream
- 1 tablespoon(14 grams) of margarine
- Salt and pepper to taste
- 1 wiener patty

Procedures
In a little bowl, whisk the eggs, weighty cream, salt and pepper. Add spread to a dish over medium-low intensity and pour in the egg blend. When the edges of the eggs begin to set, use a spatula to push the eggs from one side to another and separate the curds. Go on until the eggs are generally cooked and remove from heat. Cook the wiener patty in a skillet over medium intensity and serve close to fried eggs.

9. Low carb pancakes
Ingredients
- 2 eggs
- 2 ounces(57 grams) of cream cheddar
- 1- 2 dippers(2- 4 grams) of stevia
- 1 teaspoon(5 mL) of vanilla concentrate
- 2 haze ladles(30 mL) of olive oil

Procedures

Add the seasoning to a blender or food processor and grind until smooth. Heat a vessel over medium intensity and add the olive oil. Pour1/ 4 of the stevia into the skillet and cook for 2- 3 beats, until brilliant. Flip and cook for 1 moment, or until the posterior side is brilliant. Top with margarine, with sugar jam, new berries, or yogurt.

10. Breakfast salad
Ingredients
- 2 mugs(60 grams) of spinach
- 2 hard- boiled eggs
- 1 ounce(28 grams) of mozzarella
- 1 Roma tomato, diced
- a big part of an avocado, cut

- haze ladles(30 mL) of olive
- 1 tablespoon(15 mL) of juice
- Salt and pepper to taste

Procedures

Add the spinach to a coliseum and subcaste with the eggs, mozzarella, tomatoes, and avocados. To make the dressing, whisk the olive oil with juice and a hint of salt and pepper. Shower the dressing over the plate of mixed flora and serve.

Chapter 5. lunch

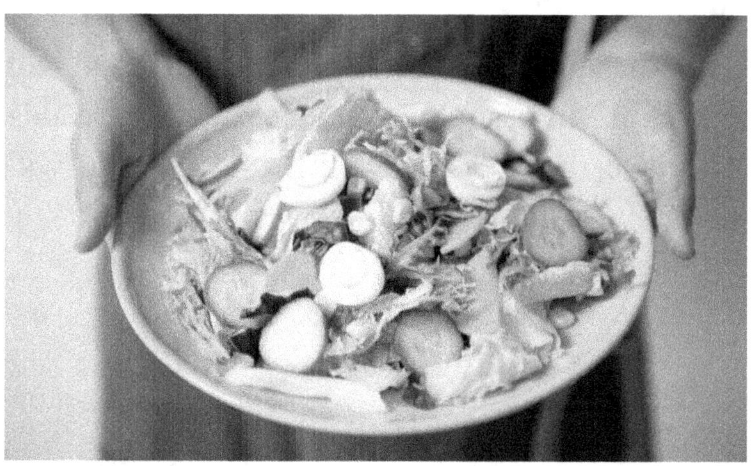

1 Cold sesame cucumber polls
Ingredients

- 1 teaspoon sesame oil
- 3 soup spoons soy sauce
- 3 soup spoons rice ginger
- 3 soup spoons tahini
- 1 tablespoon sriracha(or further according to taste)
- 1 teaspoon diced gusto
- 1 diced garlic clove
- 3 cucumbers

Procedures

A. cut into polls with a spiralizer or Y- shaped bobby ,add 8 ounces marinated warmed tofu, drained, dried, and cut into lower pieces,make 5 holes In a little coliseum, whisk together the sesame oil, soy sauce, rice ginger, tahini, sriracha, gusto and garlic.

 B. In a coliseum, set up the cucumber poles, tofu and dressing. Enhance with the scallions and sesame seeds.

2 Chicken Meatballs with Coconut-Flavor Sauce

Ingredients

MEATBALLS

- Nonstick shower
- 1 tablespoon extra-virgin olive oil
- ½ red onion
- 2 garlic cloves, minced
- 1 pound ground chicken
- ¼ cup hacked new parsley
- 1 tablespoon Dijon mustard
- ¾ teaspoon valid salt

- ½ teaspoon as of late ground faint pepper

SAUCE
- One 14-ounce could coconut whenever milk
- 1¼ cups hacked new parsley, divided
- 4 scallions, overall hacked
- 1 garlic clove, stripped and crushed
- Punch and crush of 1 lemon
- Credible salt and ground dull pepper
- Crushed red pepper chips, for serving
- 1 recipe Cauliflower Rice, for serving (discretionary)

Direction

A. MAKE THE MEATBALLS: Preheat the broiler to 375°F. Line a baking sheet with aluminum foil and give it nonstick sprinkle.

B. Heat the olive oil in a medium skillet on medium heat. Add the onion and sauté until delicate, something like 5 minutes. Add the garlic and sauté until fragrant, something like 1 second.

C. Move the onion and garlic to a medium bowl and cool reasonably. Add the mustard, parsley, and chicken; Add salt and pepper to taste. Structure the blend into around 2 tablespoon-size balls and move to the set up baking sheet. Heat the meatballs until firm and completely cooked (an inner temperature of 165°F), 17 to 20 minutes.

D. MAKE THE SAUCE: In the meantime, in the bowl of a food processor, join the coconut milk, parsley, scallions, garlic, lemon punch and lemon press and cycle until smooth; season to taste with salt and pepper.

E. Sprinkle the extra parsley and red pepper flakes over the meatballs. Serve over cauliflower rice (or one more grain or starch) showered with the sauce...

3 Potato salad

Fixings

- 50g pecans, toasted and generally cleaved
- 2 apples 1 lemon, squeezed
- 100g mayonnaise
- 2 tbsp Greek-style yogurt

- ½ tbsp Dijon mustard
- 150g red grapes, divided
- 3 celery sticks, finely cut
- 1 romaine or Little Jewel lettuce, leaves isolated and torn if huge

Procedures

Stage 1

Heat a dry griddle over a medium-high intensity and toast the pecans for 3-4 mins until delicately brilliant and sweet-smelling. Tip into a bowl and pass on to cool.

Stage 2

Throw the apples with a sprinkle of the lemon juice to forestall them staining. Join the mayonnaise, yogurt, mustard and remaining lemon juice in a huge bowl and season well. The dressing will keep chilled for as long as two days. Blend the apples, grapes and celery with the dressing and throw well in an enormous bowl to guarantee everything is uniformly covered. Orchestrate the lettuce leaves on a serving platter and spoon over the apple blend and any leftover dressing from the bowl.

Dissipate over the toasted pecans prior to serving.

4. Cold Sesame Cucumber Noodles
Ingredients
- 1 tablespoon sesame oil
- 3 tablespoons soy sauce
- 3 tablespoons rice vinegar
- 3 tablespoons tahini
- 1 teaspoon sriracha (or more to taste)
- 1 tablespoon minced ginger
- 1 garlic clove, minced
- 3 cucumbers, cut into noodles with a spiralizer or Y-formed peeler
- 8-ounce bundle marinated heated tofu — depleted, dried and cut into scaled down pieces
- 5 scallions, daintily cut
- ¼ teaspoon sesame seeds, toasted

Directions

A. In a little bowl, whisk together the sesame oil, soy sauce, rice vinegar, tahini, sriracha, ginger and garlic.

B. In an enormous bowl, throw together the cucumber noodles, tofu and dressing. Decorate with the scallions and sesame seeds.

5. Zucchini and Tomato Ragù
Fixings

- 6 tablespoons extra-virgin olive oil
- 1 onion, stripped and generally slashed
- 2 garlic cloves, stripped and softly squashed
- 1 medium zucchini, cut
- 1 medium summer squash, cut
- Genuine salt and newly ground dark pepper
- 7 ounces ready, tasty tomatoes, cleaved
- 4 ounces mozzarella, generally torn
- ¼ cup parsley leaves, generally cleaved
- ¼ cup basil leaves, torn

Directions

A. Heat the oil in a huge non-stick skillet over medium intensity. Add the onion and garlic and cook, mixing frequently, until the onion is clear, 8 to 10 minutes.

B. Add the zucchini and summer squash; season with salt and pepper. Cook, mixing every now and again, until the zucchini and summer sauce become brilliant, around 2 minutes.

C. Mix in the tomatoes and cook until they have quite recently become relaxed and the zucchini and summer squash are still somewhat firm, around 2 minutes. Serve finished off with the mozzarella, parsley and basil.

6. Tomato Salad with Barbecued Halloumi

Fixings

- 1 pound tomatoes, cut into adjusts
- ½ lemon
- Flaky salt and newly ground pepper
- Extra-virgin olive oil
- ½ pound halloumi cheddar, cut into 4 chunks
- 5 basil leaves, torn
- 2 tablespoons finely cleaved level leaf parsley

Directions

A. Preheat a barbecue or barbecue container over medium-high intensity.

B. Organize the tomatoes on a serving platter or four plates. Gently press the lemon over them and season with flaky salt and pepper.

C. Brush the barbecue grates with oil, then, at that point, add the halloumi and cook, turning once, until marks show up and the cheddar is warmed all through, around 1 moment for every side. Put on top of the tomatoes. Shower the plate of mixed greens with olive oil and sprinkle with the basil and parsley. Serve right away.

7. Greek Yogurt Chicken Plate of mixed greens Stuffed Peppers

Fixings

- ⅔ cup Greek yogurt
- 2 tablespoons Dijon mustard
- 2 tablespoons prepared rice vinegar
- Salt and newly ground dark pepper
- ⅓ cup hacked new parsley
- Meat from 1 rotisserie chicken, cubed
- 4 stems celery, cut
- 1 pack scallions, cut and isolated

- 1 16 ounces cherry tomatoes, quartered and partitioned
- ½ English cucumber, diced
- 3 chime peppers, split and seeds removed

Directions

A. In a medium bowl, whisk together the Greek yogurt, mustard and rice vinegar; season to taste with salt and pepper. Mix in the parsley.

B. Add the chicken, celery and 3/4 every one of the scallions, tomatoes and cucumbers. Mix well to join.

C. Split the chicken serving of mixed greens between the ringer pepper boats; embellish with the leftover scallions, tomatoes and cucumbers.

8. Chicken and Snap Pea Mix Fry
Ingredients
- ⅔ cup Greek yogurt
- 2 tablespoons Dijon mustard
- 2 tablespoons prepared rice vinegar
- Salt and newly ground dark pepper
- ⅓ cup hacked new parsley
- Meat from 1 rotisserie chicken, cubed

- 4 stems celery, cut
- 1 pack scallions, cut and isolated
- 1 16 ounces cherry tomatoes, quartered and separated
- ½ English cucumber, diced
- 3 toll peppers, separated and seeds removed

Directions

A. In a medium bowl, whisk together the Greek yogurt, mustard and rice vinegar; season to taste with salt and pepper. Blend in the parsley.

B. Add the chicken, celery and 3/4 all of the scallions, tomatoes and cucumbers. Blend well to join.

C. Part the chicken serving of leafy greens between the ringer pepper boats; adorn with the abundance scallions, tomatoes and cucumbers.

9. Little Eggplant Pizzas

Ingredients

- 1 large (or 2 medium) eggplants
- ⅓ cup olive oil
- Salt and recently ground dim pepper

- 1¼ cups marinara sauce
- 1½ cups obliterated mozzarella cheddar
- 2 cups cherry tomatoes, split
- ½ cup torn basil leaves

Directions

A. Preheat the oven to 400°F. Line a baking sheet with material paper.

B. Remove the completions of the eggplant(s) and a short time later cut into ¾-inch-thick cuts. Coordinate the cuts on the set up baking sheets and brush the different sides of each cut with olive oil. Season with salt and pepper.

C. Cook the eggplant cuts until practically fragile, 10 to 12 minutes.

D. Remove the plate from the oven and spread 2 tablespoons of marinara sauce on top of each piece. Top generously with mozzarella and arrange 3 to 5 cherry tomato pieces on top of each.

E. Return the pizzas to the broiler and cook for another 5 to 7 minutes, or until the tomatoes are mushy and the cheddar has melted.

F. Serve the pizzas hot, decorated with basil.

10. Cold Lemon Zoodles
Ingredients
- 1 lemon, zested and pressed
- ½ teaspoon Dijon mustard
- ½ teaspoon garlic powder
- ⅓ cup olive oil
- Salt and recently ground dull pepper
- 3 medium zucchini, cut into noodles
- 1 pack radishes, gently cut
- 1 tablespoon separated new thyme

Directions
A. In a little bowl, whisk the lemon punch, lemon juice, mustard and garlic powder to combine.

B. Step by step add the olive oil and speed to solidify. Season with salt and pepper.

C. In a gigantic bowl, toss the zucchini noodles with the radishes. Add the dressing and toss until the veggies are especially covered.

D. Serve immediately, enlivened with new thyme.

Chapter 6. Dinner

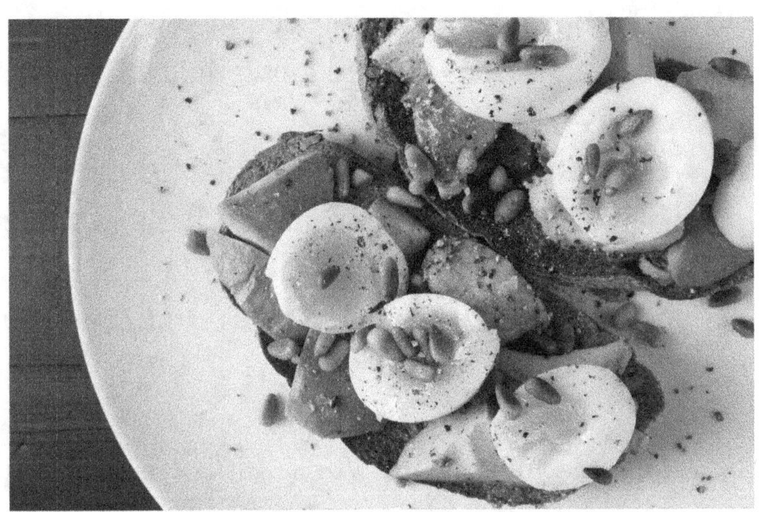

1. Chicken and Snap Pea Mix Fry
Ingredients
- 2 tablespoons vegetable oil
- 1 bundle scallions, daintily cut
- 2 garlic cloves, minced
- 1 red ringer pepper, daintily cut
- 2½ cups snap peas
- 1¼ cups boneless skinless chicken bosom,cut
- Salt and newly ground dark pepper
- 3 tablespoons soy sauce or tamari

- 2 tablespoons rice vinegar
- 2 teaspoons Sriracha (discretionary)
- 2 tablespoons sesame seeds
- 3 tablespoons hacked new cilantro

Directions

A. In a sauté skillet, heat the oil over medium intensity. Add the scallions and garlic, and sauté until fragrant, around 1 moment. Add the ringer pepper and snap peas, and sauté until simply delicate, 2 to 3 minutes.

B. Add the chicken and cook until it is brilliant and completely cooked and the vegetables are delicate, 4 to 5 minutes.

C. Add the soy sauce, rice vinegar, Sriracha (if utilizing) and sesame seeds; throw well to join. Permit the combination to stew for 1 to 2 minutes.

D. Mix in the cilantro, then embellish with a sprinkle of additional cilantro and sesame seeds. Serve right away.

2. Shrimp Scampi Zoodles

Fixings

- 2 tablespoons unsalted spread
- 2 tablespoons extra-virgin olive oil
- 3 garlic cloves
- Zing and juice of 1 lemon
- ⅓ cup dry white wine
- 1½ pounds huge tail-on shrimp, stripped
- Salt and newly ground dark pepper
- 3 pounds zucchini, spiralized
- Lemon wedges, depending on the situation for serving
- ⅓ cup hacked new parsley

Directions

A. In a huge skillet, liquefy the margarine over medium intensity. Add the olive oil and garlic; cook until fragrant, 1 moment.

B. Add the lemon zing, lemon squeeze and wine; bring to a stew. Stew until the fluid is totally decreased, around 3 minutes.

C. Add the shrimp and sauté until recently cooked, around 3 minutes. Season with salt and pepper. Move to a bowl.

D. Add the spiralized zucchini to the dish and season with salt and pepper. Cook, throwing periodically, until delicate, around 5 minutes. Return the shrimp to the skillet and throw to consolidate.

E. Serve right away, decorated with lemon and parsley.

3. Bruschetta Chicken
Fixings
- 4 meager cut boneless, skinless chicken bosoms
- Fit salt and newly ground dark pepper
- 2 teaspoons garlic powder
- 1 tablespoon Italian flavoring
- 3 tablespoons extra-virgin olive oil, partitioned

- 4 medium tomatoes, diced
- ½ red onion, minced
- 2 garlic cloves, minced
- ⅓ cup new cleaved new basil
- Balsamic vinegar, for wrapping up
- Ground Parmesan cheddar, for finishing

Directions

A. Season the chicken on the two sides with salt, pepper, garlic powder and Italian flavoring.

B. Heat 2 tablespoons of the olive oil in an enormous skillet over medium intensity. Add the chicken to the container and cook until all around sautéed on the two sides and completely cooked, 8 to 10 minutes.

C. While the chicken cooks, combine as one the leftover 1 tablespoon olive oil, tomatoes, red onion, garlic and basil.

D. Split the tomato blend between the chicken bosoms, putting a major scoop on top. Embellish with extra basil, balsamic vinegar and Parmesan. Serve right away.

4. Zucchini Pizza Dish

Fixings

- 4 cups destroyed unpeeled zucchini
- 1/2 teaspoon salt
- 2 huge eggs
- 1/2 cup ground Parmesan cheddar
- 2 cups destroyed part-skim mozzarella cheddar, separated
- 1 cup destroyed cheddar, separated
- 1 pound ground hamburger
- 1/2 cup slashed onion
- 1 can (15 ounces) Italian pureed tomatoes
- 1 medium green or sweet red pepper, slashed

Procedures

A. Preheat the boiler to 400°. Place zucchini in a colander; sprinkle with salt. Let stand for 10 minutes, then crush out dampness.

B. Join zucchini with eggs, Parmesan and around 50% of the mozzarella and cheddar cheeses. Press into a lubed 13x9-in. or then again 3-qt. baking dish. Heat for 20 minutes.

C. In the meantime, in an enormous pan, cook hamburger and onion over medium intensity until meat is presently not pink, breaking meat into disintegrates; channel. Add pureed tomatoes; spoon over zucchini combination. Sprinkle with residual cheeses; add green pepper. Prepare until warmed through, around 20 minutes longer.

5. Zesty Lemon-Ginger Chicken Soup
Fixings
- One 4-pound entire chicken, innards removed
- 1 huge yellow onion, stripped and slashed into enormous pieces

- 2 medium carrots, cleaved into enormous pieces
- 2 celery stems, cleaved into enormous pieces
- 1 big head garlic, cut transversely
- ½ to 1 jalapeño, cut longwise
- Two 3-inch pieces ginger, stripped and cleaved
- 1 enormous bundle new parsley
- 1 tablespoon coriander seeds
- 1 tablespoon fit salt
- 2 teaspoons newly ground dark pepper
- 6 ounces new spinach or other delicate greens
- 2 lemons, meagerly sliced

Directions

A. Join the chicken, onion, carrot, celery, garlic, jalapeño, ginger, parsley, coriander, salt and dark pepper in an enormous Dutch stove or pot. Add sufficient virus water to cover. Cover the pot and heat the fluid to the point of boiling over high intensity, then, at that point, decrease the intensity to low and stew, skimming any pollutants that could ascend to the highest point of the fluid with a metal spoon. Cover and stew until the chicken is delicate and goes to pieces, 55 minutes to 60 minutes. (On the other hand, you can cook the chicken and stock in a strain cooker for 40 minutes.)

B. Move the chicken to a huge plate and gather any stock that could trickle down. Utilizing a fine-network sifter, strain the stock into a perfect pan and keep warm over low intensity. Taste the stock and add salt assuming you feel it needs it. Shred the chicken using a fork. Assuming you have more meat than you might want to serve, this is perfect to freeze for another utilization.

C. Partition the spinach, destroyed chicken, jalapeño and lemon cuts among serving bowls and top with the hot stock.

6. Chicken Wings
Fixings
- BAGEL Preparing
- 2 tablespoons poppy seeds
- 2 tablespoons sesame seeds

- 1 tablespoon dried onion pieces
- 2 teaspoons coarse Himalayan pink salt
- 1 teaspoon dried minced garlic
- 3 pounds chicken wings, managed and isolated into wingettes and drumettes
- 3 tablespoons spread, dissolved
- 3 tablespoons All that Bagel Preparing

Procedures

A. Preheat the broiler to 400°F.

B. Put the poppy seeds, sesame seeds, onion drops, salt and garlic in a little bowl and blend well. The flavoring can be put away in a water/air proof compartment for as long as 90 days

C. MAKE THE CHICKEN WINGS: Spread the chicken wing pieces in a solitary layer on a baking sheet. Prepare until the wings are brilliant and firm, 40 to 45 minutes. Eliminate from the stove and move the wings to a serving bowl.

D. Pour the liquefied spread over the wings, then mix or throw to cover the wings in the margarine. Sprinkle all that bagel preparing over the wings and shake to equitably cover them.

NOTE: Store extras in an impermeable holder in the cooler for as long as 5 days. To warm, heat 2 tablespoons of avocado oil in a huge skillet over medium intensity. Add the wings and cook until fresh and warmed through, around 2 minutes for each side.

7. Skillet Pepper Steak
Fixings

- 12 ounces top round meat, daintily cut
- Genuine salt and newly ground dark pepper
- 2 tablespoons nut oil (or other nonpartisan oil), separated
- 1 tablespoon soy sauce
- 1 tablespoon rice wine vinegar
- 1½ teaspoons crushed red-pepper pieces
- 1 red chime pepper, meagerly cut
- 1 yellow chime pepper, meagerly cut

- 1 green chime pepper, meagerly cut
- 1 orange chime pepper, meagerly cut
- 3 garlic cloves, minced
- 1 pack scallions, meagerly cut
- Sesame seeds, depending on the situation for wrapping up

Procedures

A. Season the steak with salt and pepper. In a huge skillet, heat 1 tablespoon of the oil over medium-high intensity. Add the steak to the skillet and pan fried food until caramelized on the outside however not completely cooked, around 2 minutes.

B. Move the steak to a medium bowl. Add the soy sauce, rice wine vinegar and crushed red-pepper pieces. Throw well to join.

C. In a similar skillet, heat the excess 1 tablespoon oil over medium intensity. Add the peppers in an even layer. Cook, throwing once in a while, until simply delicate, around 4 minutes.

D. Push the peppers aside of the skillet and return the steak to the opposite side of the skillet. Cook for 2 minutes. Mix the garlic into the peppers and cook for a brief time.

E. Embellish the steak with scallions and sesame seeds. Serve right away.

8. Honey-Mustard Sheet Container Salmon Fixings

- 1 tablespoon light-shaded crude honey
- 1 tablespoon coarse-grain mustard
- ½ teaspoon white wine vinegar
- Fine ocean salt and newly ground dark pepper
- One (2-pound) salmon filet, pin bones removed
- 2½ cups stripped, cultivated, and cubed butternut squash
- 12 ounces Brussels grows, managed and split

- 2 cups cherry tomatoes
- 2 tablespoons avocado oil or liquefied ghee
- ½ teaspoon newly crushed lemon juice
- ¼ teaspoon garlic powder
- ¼ teaspoon onion powder
- ¾ teaspoon dried oregano, separated
- ⅛ teaspoon ground turmeric
- 1 lemon, daintily cut transversely

Procedures

A. In a little bowl, whisk together the honey, mustard, vinegar, ½ teaspoon of the oregano, ½ teaspoon salt and ¼ teaspoon pepper.Place the salmon filet in a baking dish and pour the marinade over the fish. Marinate for 15 minutes.

B. Preheat the stove to 400°F.

C. In the meantime, in a huge bowl, throw together the butternut squash, Brussels sprouts, tomatoes, oil, lemon juice, garlic powder, onion powder, remaining ¼ teaspoon oregano, turmeric, ¼ teaspoon salt and ⅛ teaspoon pepper. Spread the vegetables around the edges of a huge rimmed baking sheet.

D. Eliminate the salmon from the marinade, permitting any overabundance to dribble once more into the baking dish. Save the marinade. Place the salmon in the focal point of the baking sheet and orchestrate the lemon cuts on top of the fish.

E. Cook until the fish drops in the middle and the vegetables are fresh delicate, brushing the fish with the held marinade like clockwork, 16 to 18 minutes..

9. Paleo Egg Roll in a Bowl
Fixings
- 1½ tablespoons sesame oil
- 3 carrots, stripped and destroyed
- ¼ head red cabbage, destroyed
- ¼ head green cabbage, destroyed

- 1 bundle scallions, cut on the predisposition
- 2 garlic cloves, minced
- 1 tablespoon minced ginger
- 1 pound ground pork
- 2 tablespoons soy sauce or tamari
- 1½ tablespoons unseasoned rice vinegar
- 1 tablespoon sriracha
- Sesame seeds, cilantro leaves and meagerly cut red chiles, for serving

Procedures

A. In a medium skillet, heat the oil over medium intensity. Add the carrots, red and green cabbage, and cook until delicate, around 3 minutes.

B. Add the scallions, garlic and ginger and cook until fragrant, around 1 moment. Add the pork and sauté until completely cooked and presently not pink, 6 to 7 minutes.

C. Season the combination with the soy sauce, rice vinegar and sriracha. Serve finished off with sesame seeds, cilantro and red chiles.

10. Salmon with Pesto and Rankled Tomatoes
Fixings
- 1 pound blended cherry tomatoes
- 3 garlic cloves, minced
- Fit salt and newly ground dark pepper
- 3 tablespoons extra-virgin olive oil
- 1 large (1 to 1½ pounds) focus cut salmon filet or 4 little filets (3 to 4 ounces each)
- 1 cup basil pesto (locally acquired or custom made)

Procedures

A. Preheat the broiler to 425°F. Line a baking sheet with material paper.

B. On the baking sheet, throw together the cherry tomatoes, garlic and a sprinkle of salt and pepper. Heat until the tomatoes have exploded and are somewhat seared, 15 to 16 minutes.

C. Line a different baking sheet with material paper for the salmon. Brush a light layer of olive oil onto the fillet(s) and season with salt and pepper.

D. Prepare for 10 minutes, then spoon 1 to 2 tablespoons of the pesto equally over the salmon. Prepare until the salmon chips off effectively when pushed with a fork, around 3 minutes more.

E. Tenderly exchange the salmon to a serving platter and top with the burst tomatoes.

NOTE: On the off chance that you don't like salmon, you can supplant it with cod or halibut.

Chapter 7. Snacks

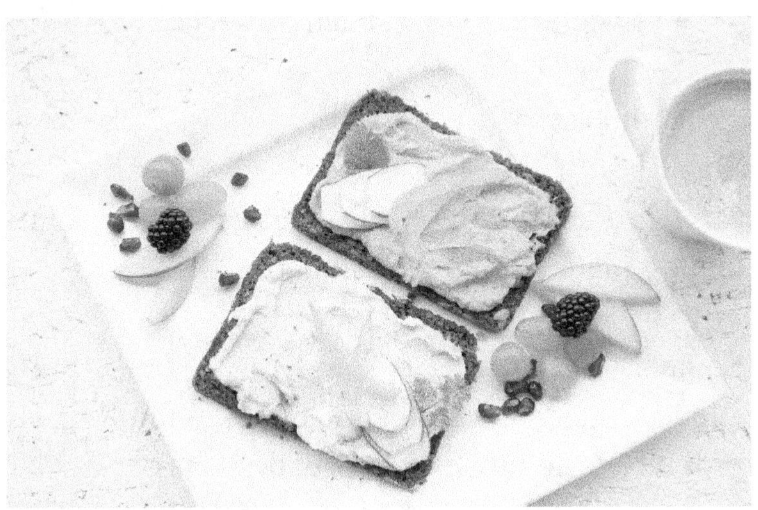

1. Nutty chicken satay strips
Fixings
- 2 tbsp thick peanut butter (without palm oil or sugar)
- 1 garlic clove, finely ground
- 1 tsp Madras curry powder
- hardly any shakes soy sauce
- 2 tsp lime juice

- 2 skinless, chicken bosom filets (around 300g) cut into thick strips
- around 10cm cucumber, cut into fingers
- sweet bean stew sauce, to serve

Procedures

Stage 1

Heat broiler to 200C/180C fan/gas 4 and line a baking plate with non-stick paper.

Stage 2

Blend 2 tbsp thick peanut butter with 1 finely ground garlic clove, 1 tsp Madras curry powder, a couple of shakes of soy sauce and 2 tsp lime juice in a bowl. Some nut spreads are thicker than others, so if essential, add a hint of bubbling water to get a covering consistency.

Stage 3

Add 2 skinless chicken bosom filets, cut into strips, and blend well. Orchestrate on the baking sheet, separated, and prepare in the broiler for 8-10 mins until cooked, yet succulent.

2. Aubergine and chickpea chomps
Fixings

- 3 huge aubergines, divided, cut side scored
- splash oil
- 2 fat garlic cloves, stripped
- 2 tsp coriander
- 2 tsp cumin seeds
- 400g can chickpeas, depleted
- 2 tbsp gram flour
- 1 lemon, ½ zested and squeeze, ½ slice into wedges to serve (discretionary)
- 3 tbsp polenta
- For the plunge
- 1 tbsp harissa
- 150g coconut sans dairy yogurt

Procedures
Stage 1

Heat broiler to 200C/180C fan/gas 6. Shower the aubergine parts liberally with oil, then, at that point, set them cut-side up in an enormous broiling tin with the garlic, coriander and cumin seeds. Season, then broil for 40 mins until the aubergine is totally delicate. Put away to cool a bit.

Stage 2

Scoop the aubergine tissue into a bowl and dispose of the skins. Utilize a spatula to scratch the flavors and garlic into the bowl. Add the chickpeas, gram flour, lemon zing and juice, generally squash together and really look at the flavoring. You can definitely relax in the event that the blend is a delicate piece - it will solidify in the ice chest.

3. Melon with mint and feta
Fixings

- 2 x 5cm wedges of watermelon
- 40g feta, disintegrated
- modest bunch hacked mint
- 2 wedges of lime

Procedures

Stage 1

Take each wedge of melon and cut between the skin and tissue to isolate them, then, at that point, slice downwards to make scaled down lumps. Flick out the seeds, disperse over the feta and mint, and crush over the lime prior to serving.

4. Omelet roll-up

Fixings

- 1 egg
- a little rapeseed or olive oil for broiling
- 2 tbsp tomato salsa
- around 1 tbsp new coriander

Procedures

Stage 1

Beat the egg with 1 tbsp water. Heat the oil in a medium non-stick container. Add the egg and twirl round the foundation of the dish, like you are making a flapjack, and cook until set. There is a compelling reason I need to turn it in.

Stage 2

Carefully tip the hotcake onto a board, spread with the salsa, sprinkle with the coriander, then, at that point, roll it up. It tends to be eaten warm or cold - you can save it for 2 days in the refrigerator.

5. Sound fish lettuce wraps
Fixings

- 2 drops rapeseed oil, for brushing
- 2 x 140g new fish filets, thawed out
- 1 ready avocado
- ½ tsp English mustard powder
- 1 tsp juice vinegar
- 1 tbsp tricks
- 8 romaine lettuce leaves
- 16 cherry tomatoes, ideally on the plant, split

Procedures

Stage 1

Brush the fish with just enough oil. Heat a non-stick dish, add the fish and cook for 1 min each side, or a min or so longer for a thicker filet. Move to a plate to rest.

Stage 2

Split and stone the avocado and scoop the tissue into a little bowl. Add the mustard powder and vinegar, then, at that point, pound well so the combination is smooth like mayonnaise. Mix in the escapades. Spoon into two little dishes and place on serving plates with the lettuce leaves, and tomatoes.

6. Peppery fennel and carrot salad
Fixings

- 2 big carrots, cut into dainty sticks or ground
- 2 big fennel bulbs, quartered and daintily cut

- modest bunch nut or cashew nuts, hacked
- 2 tbsp olive oil
- 1 tsp mustard seed
- 1 tsp nigella or dark onion seeds (discretionary)
- juice 1 lemon or lime

Procedures

Stage 1

Tip the carrots and fennel into a plate of mixed greens bowl. Toast the nuts in a hot skillet for 3-5 mins until brilliant, then tip onto a plate. In a similar skillet, heat the oil and sear the mustard and nigella or dark onion seeds, if utilizing, until they start to pop - around 30 secs. Pour in the lemon or lime squeeze and combine as one to make a dressing. Throw along with the vegetables in the bowl, then sprinkle with nuts to serve.

7. Amalfi servings of mixed greens

Fixings

- 50g pine nut
- 2 x 110g packs salad leaves (we utilized bistro salad with red chard)
- 200g SunBlush tomato, generally slashed
- 200g dark olive (niçoise are perfect)

For the dressing

- 1 tbsp sundried tomato glue
- 1 tbsp balsamic vinegar
- 5 tbsp olive oil

Procedures

Stage 1

The other day, I made the dressing. Blend the tomato glue and vinegar in a little bowl. Gradually rush in the olive oil to frame a smooth emulsion and season to taste. Store it in a screw-top container to excel and re-whisk prior to utilizing in the evening.

Stage 2

The pine nuts can be managed the day preceding to save time. Heat a little skillet, tip in the nuts and cook for 2-3 minutes, turning them much of the time until they smell nutty and are well caramelized.

8. Watermelon salsa

Fixings

- 200g watermelon
- 2 little shallots
- little bundle coriander
- juice 1/2 lime
- 2 tbsp olive oil

Procedures

Stage 1

Finely cleave 200g watermelon, 2 little shallots and a little pack coriander. Combine as one with juice ½ lime and 2 tbsp olive oil. Season and act as a plunge or heap on top of messy nachos.

9. Chicory and hummus nibbles

Fixings

- 2 enormous heads of chicory
- 1 carrot
- 175g tub hummus
- 16-18 dark olives, ideally hollowed

Procedures

Stage 1

Up to 2 hrs ahead, separate the chicory into boat-formed departures and trim the closures with the goal that they are generally a similar size. You will presumably get around eight or nine good measured leaves from each head of chicory. As the leaves draw nearer to the core of the chicory, they will be too little to even think about utilizing for canapés, so save them to add to stormy servings of mixed greens.

Stage 2

Strip the carrot, then continue to strip off strips until you have as numerous as the quantity of chicory leaves.

Stage 3

Drop spoonfuls of hummus onto the chicory, then, at that point, add a carrot twist and an olive to each. They'll be stored in the refrigerator for around 2 hours.

10. Zesty cheddar nibbles
Fixings
- 85g plain flour
- 50g spread, slashed
- 50g mature gruyère, ground
- 25g new parmesan (or veggie lover elective), finely ground
- 2 eggs, all around beaten
- 1l vegetable oil, for profound broiling

Procedures

Stage 1

Filter the flour and some salt into a bowl. Set a non-leave dish on the intensity with 150ml virus water and the cleaved spread. Bring to the bubble, blending until the spread melts. Tip in all the flour and, utilizing a wooden spoon, beat hard until the blend becomes smooth and begins to leave the side of the container.

Stage 2

Eliminate from the intensity, beat in the gruyère and around 50% of the parmesan and cool for 5 mins. Bit by bit beat in the eggs until you have a smooth, thick, however spoonable blend - you may not require all the egg. Can be saved now for 2 hrs without chilling.

Stage 3

At the point when prepared to serve, heat the oil in a profound fat skillet to around 180C. Utilizing 2 teaspoons gather up flawless bits and cautiously drop into the hot oil. Broil 6-8 dabs a

period for 3-4 mins until brilliant and fresh -
dunk the bits under to equally brown. Warm the
oil as needs be. Channel on paper towels,
sprinkle with the remainder of the parmesan.
Serve hot.

Chapter 8. FAQs

Is the Galveston diet equivalent to keto's?

No, it isn't. While the two weight control plans center around a high-fat, low-carb diet, the Galveston diet incorporates an exceptionally low-carb diet stacked with calming feasts eaten inside a 8-hour time span.

Is Galveston a purgative?

No, the eating routine spotlights on lessening weight through adjusting your hormonal levels as opposed to helping solid discharges.

Is the Galveston diet better compared to the Mediterranean eating regimen?

There is no definitive proof recommending that the Galveston diet is superior to the Mediterranean eating regimen. The two eating regimens follow a comparable standard of including mitigating food sources. In any case, the previous additionally incorporates 16/8 discontinuous fasting and is somewhat more prohibitive.

Is the Galveston diet sound?
Wellbeing and nourishment specialists say the eating regimen can be solid. "The accentuation on restricting excessively handled food varieties, and empowering products of the soil is somewhat positive,""The diet is sound since it suggests removing and restricting handled food varieties, added sugar, and other counterfeit fixings,"

Would it be a good idea for me to attempt to eat less carbs?
It's essential to make lifestyle changes when you hit menopause. Ladies should know that on the off chance that they don't change something at menopause — eat less and practice more — they will put on weight.

What are the 4 things to follow on the Galveston diet

you ought to follow fiber, vitamin D, Omega 3, unsaturated fats, and magnesium. After you track them for seven days, I believe that you should pick sustenance. that will raise those qualities to 100 percent of the RDA. Try not to count calories, don't count macros.